BRANDON DEMARTINIS

Fitpreneur's Handbook

Dynamic Full Body Workouts for Success-Driven Entrepreneurs

No man has the right to be an amateur in
the matter of physical training. It is a shame
for a man to grow old without seeing the
beauty and strength of which his body is
capable.

SOCRATES

Contents

1

The Fitpreneur Mindset

Entrepreneurship is an exhilarating journey filled with opportunities, growth, and challenges. As an entrepreneur, your days are often consumed by the demands of building and managing a business. In this fast-paced environment, it's easy to overlook your personal well-being, particularly your physical fitness. However, maintaining a healthy lifestyle is crucial not only for your personal well-being but also for your business success. In this chapter, we will delve into the unique challenges faced by entrepreneurs in maintaining a healthy lifestyle, discuss the importance of cultivating a mindset that prioritizes both fitness and business success, and explore the benefits of integrating exercise into your entrepreneurial journey.

Understanding the Challenges

Entrepreneurs face a set of unique challenges that can make it difficult to maintain a healthy lifestyle. Long working hours, high levels of stress, and constant decision-making can take a toll on physical and mental health. The pressure to meet deadlines, secure funding, and compete in a rapidly changing market can lead to neglecting self-care habits such as exercise and healthy eating.

Moreover, the blurred boundaries between work and personal life can make it challenging to carve out time for fitness. Entrepreneurs often find themselves constantly connected, answering emails and attending to business matters even during their supposed downtime. This lack of separation can lead to a sedentary lifestyle and increased stress levels, further exacerbating the challenges to maintaining a healthy routine.

Cultivating the Fitpreneur Mindset

To overcome these challenges, it's essential to cultivate a mindset that prioritizes both fitness and business success. The fitpreneur mindset acknowledges that physical health is not separate from business success but rather a crucial component of it. Here are some key principles to consider:

1. Mindfulness: Develop self-awareness and be mindful of the impact your lifestyle choices have on your well-being. Recognize that neglecting your physical health can have negative consequences for your business in the long run. Make a conscious decision to prioritize fitness as an integral part of your entrepreneurial journey.

2. Goal Setting: Set clear fitness goals just as you would set goals for your business. Whether it's completing a marathon or improving your strength and stamina, having specific fitness goals helps to provide direction and motivation. Break these goals down into manageable steps and track your progress regularly.

3. Time Management: Efficiently manage your time by creating a schedule that incorporates dedicated time for exercise. Treat exercise as a non-negotiable appointment and block out time on your calendar accordingly. By proactively managing your time, you can strike a balance between work and fitness.

4. Accountability: Find ways to hold yourself accountable for your fitness commitments. This could involve partnering with a workout buddy, hiring a personal trainer, or joining a fitness

community. Surrounding yourself with like-minded individuals who understand the demands of entrepreneurship can provide support and motivation.

Benefits of Exercise for Entrepreneurs

Integrating exercise into your entrepreneurial journey offers a multitude of benefits. Let's explore some of the ways in which exercise positively impacts both your personal well-being and business success:

1. Improved Energy and Productivity: Regular exercise boosts energy levels, enhances cognitive function, and increases productivity. Engaging in physical activity releases endorphins, educes stress hormones, and promotes better sleep. These factors contribute to improved focus, creativity, and overall mental well-being, enabling you to tackle business challenges with clarity and vigor.

2. Enhanced Stress Management: The entrepreneurial journey is riddled with stress, and exercise serves as a powerful tool to combat it. Physical activity stimulates the production of neurotransmitters like serotonin and dopamine, which are known to reduce stress and improve mood. Regular exercise can help you develop effective coping mechanisms, leading to better stress management skills.

3. Increased Resilience: Entrepreneurship requires resilience in the face of setbacks and obstacles. Engaging in challenging workouts builds mental and physical resilience, translating into a stronger mindset to overcome business hurdles. The discipline and determination developed through exercise can positively influence your approach to problem-solving and decision-making.

4. Networking Opportunities: Fitness activities provide opportunities for networking and building connections outside the business realm. Participating in group classes, sports teams, or charity runs can connect you with individuals from diverse backgrounds,

expanding your network and potentially creating new business opportunities.

Conclusion

The fitpreneur mindset emphasizes the importance of maintaining a healthy lifestyle as an entrepreneur. By understanding the unique challenges faced by entrepreneurs, cultivating a mindset that prioritizes both fitness and business success, and embracing the benefits of exercise, you can create a harmonious balance between personal well-being and entrepreneurial endeavors. Remember, taking care of yourself physically and mentally is not a distraction from your business; it is an investment in your long-term success as a fitpreneur.

2

The Foundations of Full Body Fitness

When it comes to achieving full-body fitness, it's important to have a well-rounded fitness routine that addresses all key components of physical fitness. In this chapter, we will explore the essential elements of a comprehensive fitness routine, discuss the importance of setting realistic goals, and guide you through the process of assessing your current fitness level to identify areas for improvement. By understanding these foundations, you can create a personalized workout plan that will help you achieve optimal fitness.

Key Components of a Well-Rounded Fitness Routine

A well-rounded fitness routine encompasses several key components that collectively contribute to overall physical fitness. These components include:

1. Cardiovascular Endurance: Cardiovascular exercises, such as running, cycling, swimming, or aerobics, improve the health of your heart and lungs. They increase your endurance, enhance your body's ability to utilize oxygen and improve overall cardiovascular fitness.

2. Strength Training: Strength training involves using resistance,

such as weights or bodyweight exercises, to strengthen and tone your muscles. It helps build lean muscle mass, increase bone density, and improve overall strength and power. Incorporating exercises that target major muscle groups, such as squats, deadlifts, push-ups, and rows, into your routine is essential for full body strength.

3. Flexibility and Mobility: Flexibility exercises, such as stretching or yoga, promote joint mobility, increase range of motion, and improve muscle elasticity. Flexibility training helps prevent injuries, reduces muscle soreness, and enhances overall physical performance.

4. Balance and Coordination: Balance and coordination exercises, such as yoga poses, Tai Chi, or single-leg exercises, improve stability, body control, and proprioception. These exercises help prevent falls, enhance athletic performance, and support functional movements in daily activities.

Setting Realistic Goals and Creating a Personalized Workout Plan

Before embarking on a fitness journey, it's crucial to set realistic goals and develop a personalized workout plan. Here are some steps to guide you through the process:

1. Define Your Goals: Start by clearly defining your fitness goals. Are you looking to lose weight, gain muscle, improve endurance, or enhance overall fitness? Make sure your goals are specific, measurable, attainable, relevant, and time-bound (SMART goals).

2. Assess Your Time Availability: Consider your daily schedule and determine how much time you can allocate to exercise. Be realistic about the time you can commit to your workouts, keeping in mind other responsibilities and commitments.

3. Identify Your Preferences: Determine the types of exercises and

activities you enjoy. If you find joy in what you're doing, you're more likely to stick with your fitness routine. Whether it's running, swimming, dancing, or group fitness classes, choose activities that align with your interests and preferences.

4. Seek Professional Guidance: If you're new to fitness or unsure about creating a workout plan, consider consulting a fitness professional. They can assess your needs, provide guidance, and help design a personalized workout plan tailored to your goals and fitness level.

5. Plan Your Workouts: Once you have defined your goals and assessed your availability and preferences, it's time to plan your workouts. Structure your routine to include all key components of fitness, balancing cardiovascular exercises, strength training, flexibility work, and balance exercises throughout the week. Consider factors such as frequency, duration, and intensity of workouts while keeping in mind the principles of progression and recovery.

Assessing Your Current Fitness Level

Assessing your current fitness level is crucial in identifying areas for improvement and tracking your progress over time. Here are a few ways to assess your fitness level:

1. Cardiovascular Endurance: Measure your cardiovascular fitness by performing a timed run, walk, or cycle and recording the distance covered. Use standardized tests, such as the Cooper Test or the 12-minute run, to estimate your cardiovascular endurance level.

2. Strength and Muscular Endurance: Evaluate your muscular strength by performing exercises such as push-ups, squats, or planks and noting the number of repetitions you can complete with

proper form. Consider using a strength training app or consulting a fitness professional for a more accurate assessment.

3. Flexibility and Mobility: Assess your flexibility by performing stretches targeting major muscle groups, such as the hamstring stretch or shoulder stretch. Note the range of motion and any limitations you experience.

4. Balance and Coordination: Test your balance and coordination by performing exercises like the single-leg stand or the heel-to-toe walk. Take note of any difficulty maintaining balance or coordination during these exercises.

Conclusion

Building a solid foundation of full-body fitness requires addressing the key components of physical fitness, setting realistic goals, and creating a personalized workout plan. By incorporating cardiovascular endurance, strength training, flexibility, mobility work, and balance and coordination exercises into your routine, you can achieve a well-rounded fitness regimen. Remember to assess your current fitness level periodically to track progress and make necessary adjustments to your plan. By following these foundations, you'll be on your way to achieving optimal fitness and enjoying the countless benefits that come with it.

3

Fitness Essentials for the Busy Entrepreneur

As a busy entrepreneur, finding time for fitness can seem like an insurmountable challenge. However, prioritizing your physical well-being is essential for maintaining optimal performance in both your personal and professional life. In this chapter, we will explore time-saving strategies to incorporate workouts into a hectic schedule, discuss how efficient exercise routines can maximize productivity, and provide strategies for staying motivated and overcoming obstacles. By implementing these fitness essentials, you can lead a balanced and successful life as a busy entrepreneur.

Time-Saving Strategies

When time is limited, it's crucial to find efficient ways to incorporate workouts into your busy schedule. Here are some time-saving strategies:

1. High-Intensity Interval Training (HIIT): HIIT workouts involve short bursts of intense exercise followed by brief recovery periods. These workouts can be completed in a shorter amount of time compared to traditional steady-state cardio. By incorporating HIIT exercises like sprints, burpees, or jump squats, you can

maximize your calorie burn and cardiovascular fitness in a time-efficient manner.

2. Circuit Training: Circuit training involves performing a series of exercises back-to-back with minimal rest in between. By combining cardiovascular exercises with strength or bodyweight exercises, you can work multiple muscle groups and increase your heart rate simultaneously. This type of training not only saves time but also provides a full-body workout.

3. Active Breaks: Instead of sitting for prolonged periods, incorporate short bursts of activity throughout your day. Take regular breaks to perform exercises like squats, lunges, or jumping jacks. These brief bursts of movement not only contribute to your overall daily activity level but also increase energy and productivity.

4. Prioritize High-Impact Exercises: Focus on exercises that deliver the most significant benefits in the shortest amount of time. Compound exercises that work multiple muscle groups simultaneously, such as squats, deadlifts, and push-ups, provide efficient and effective workouts. By selecting exercises that target multiple areas, you can save time without compromising results.

Maximizing Productivity

Efficient exercise routines not only save time but also maximize productivity. Here's how you can make the most of your workouts:

1. Combine Exercise with Work-related Tasks: Look for opportunities to incorporate exercise into your work-related activities. For instance, you can have walking meetings, use a standing desk or stability ball instead of a traditional chair, or even perform simple exercises like stretching or light dumbbell exercises while reading or listening to business-related materials.

2. Plan and Prepare in Advance: Set aside time to plan your workouts

and prepare necessary equipment or workout clothes in advance. By eliminating the need for last-minute decision-making or searching for gear, you can seamlessly transition into your workout and maximize your exercise time.

3. Focus on Time-Efficient Exercises: Choose exercises that target multiple muscle groups and provide a full-body workout. Incorporate compound exercises like squats, lunges, rows, and push-ups that engage multiple joints and muscles simultaneously. This approach ensures that you make the most of your time and achieve a comprehensive workout.

4. Limit Distractions: Minimize distractions during your workout sessions. Put your phone on silent or airplane mode, avoid checking emails or social media, and create a dedicated space free from interruptions. This allows you to focus solely on your workout, maximizing your efficiency and mental engagement.

Staying Motivated and Overcoming Obstacles

Maintaining motivation and overcoming obstacles is crucial for sustaining a consistent fitness routine. Here are strategies to help you stay on track:

1. Set Realistic Goals: Establish realistic and achievable fitness goals that align with your busy schedule. Break your goals down into smaller milestones, celebrating each achievement along the way. This approach keeps you motivated and allows you to track your progress effectively.

2. Find Accountability and Support: Seek accountability partners or join fitness communities to stay motivated. Working out with a partner or participating in group classes provides support, encouragement, and a sense of camaraderie. Additionally, sharing your fitness journey with others helps maintain accountability and

increases motivation.

3. Schedule Your Workouts: Treat your workouts as non-negotiable appointments and schedule them in advance. Blocking out specific time slots on your calendar ensures that you allocate time for exercise and helps establish a routine. Treat these scheduled workouts as important meetings with yourself and prioritize them accordingly.

4. Adapt and Be Flexible: Recognize that your schedule as an entrepreneur may be unpredictable. Be prepared to adapt and adjust your workout plans as needed. If a long workout is not feasible, squeeze in a shorter, high-intensity session or break it into smaller bouts throughout the day. Flexibility and adaptability are key to maintaining consistency in the face of changing circumstances.

Conclusion

As a busy entrepreneur, integrating fitness into your hectic schedule may seem challenging, but it is essential for your overall well-being and productivity. By implementing time-saving strategies, maximizing efficiency, and staying motivated, you can successfully prioritize fitness in your life. Remember that every small step counts, and consistency is key. By making fitness an integral part of your routine, you can achieve a healthy and balanced lifestyle while thriving in your entrepreneurial journey.

4

Dynamic Full Body Workouts

In this chapter, we will introduce 5 diverse and effective full-body workouts specifically designed for busy entrepreneurs. These workouts are crafted to engage multiple muscle groups, maximize efficiency, and provide a comprehensive training experience. Each workout is carefully structured to target various areas of the body and can be tailored to different fitness levels. With detailed instructions, illustrations, and modifications, you'll have the tools to incorporate dynamic full-body workouts into your fitness routine.

Workout 1: HIIT Blast

This high-intensity interval training (HIIT) workout is designed to elevate your heart rate, burn calories, and improve cardiovascular fitness. Perform each exercise for 30 seconds, followed by a 15-second rest. Complete three rounds with a 1-minute rest between rounds.

1. Jumping Jacks
2. Burpees
3. Mountain Climbers
4. High Knees
5. Plank Jacks

Workout 2: Full Body Strength Circuit

This workout combines strength exercises to target major muscle groups while maintaining an elevated heart rate. Perform each exercise for 12-15 reps and complete three rounds with minimal rest between exercises.

1. Squats
2. Push-Ups
3. Lunges (alternating legs)
4. Bent-Over Rows
5. Dumbbell Shoulder Press

Workout 3: Cardio and Core Fusion

This workout integrates cardio exercises with core strengthening movements for a complete full-body workout. Perform each exercise for 45 seconds, followed by a 15-second rest. Complete three rounds with a 1-minute rest between rounds.

1. Jump Rope
2. Bicycle Crunches
3. High Plank Shoulder Taps
4. Box Jumps (or Step-Ups)
5. Russian Twists

Workout 4: Functional Fitness Circuit

This circuit focuses on functional movements that mimic real-life activities, improving strength, stability, and mobility. Perform each exercise for 10-12 reps and complete three rounds with minimal rest between exercises.

1. Deadlifts

2. Squat Jumps
3. Push Press
4. Single-Leg Romanian Deadlifts
5. Plank with Leg Lifts

Workout 5: Bodyweight Burnout

This bodyweight-only workout can be done anywhere, requiring no equipment. Perform each exercise for 45 seconds, followed by a 15-second rest. Complete three rounds with a 1-minute rest between rounds.

1. Walking Lunges
2. Push-Ups
3. Glute Bridges
4. Mountain Climbers
5. Plank Hold

Illustrations and Modifications

To ensure proper form and technique, detailed illustrations are provided for each exercise in the workout plan. These visuals serve as a reference guide, allowing you to perform the exercises correctly and minimize the risk of injury. Additionally, modifications are included to accommodate different fitness levels.

For beginners or individuals with limited mobility, modifications may include reducing the intensity or range of motion, using lighter weights, or performing alternative exercises. Intermediate and advanced fitness enthusiasts can increase the difficulty by adding resistance, increasing repetitions, or shortening rest periods.

Instructions and Progression

Each workout includes step-by-step instructions for performing the exercises, ensuring that you understand the correct form and technique.

It is essential to prioritize proper form to maximize effectiveness and reduce the risk of injury.

To progress, gradually increase the intensity or challenge of the workouts over time. This can be achieved by adding more resistance, increasing repetitions, decreasing rest periods, or incorporating advanced variations of the exercises.

Customization and Variety

While the workouts provided offer a wide range of exercises and training modalities, it's essential to customize your routine based on personal preferences and fitness goals. Feel free to mix and match exercises from different workouts, experiment with different formats, and add variety to keep your workouts exciting and engaging.

Conclusion

These 5 dynamic full-body workouts are designed to help busy entrepreneurs incorporate efficient and effective training into their schedules. By engaging multiple muscle groups, these workouts provide a comprehensive training experience that improves strength, endurance, and overall fitness. With detailed instructions, illustrations, and modifications, you have the flexibility to tailor the workouts to your fitness level and preferences. Remember to prioritize proper form, gradually progress, and add variety to your routine to maintain motivation and achieve optimal results.

5

Fitness and Mental Performance

In this chapter, we will explore the fascinating relationship between physical fitness and mental performance. While we often associate exercise with physical health, research has shown that regular physical activity can have a profound impact on cognitive function and mental well-being. In this chapter, we will examine the correlation between physical fitness and cognitive function, explore techniques to enhance mental clarity, focus, and creativity through exercise, and discuss strategies for incorporating mindfulness and stress management into your fitness routine. By understanding the connection between fitness and mental performance, you can optimize both your physical and mental well-being.

The Correlation Between Physical Fitness and Cognitive Function

Research has demonstrated a strong correlation between physical fitness and cognitive function. Engaging in regular exercise has been linked to improvements in various cognitive abilities, including attention, memory, problem-solving, and decision-making. Exercise increases blood flow to the brain, promoting the growth of new neurons and enhancing neural connectivity. It also stimulates the release of chemicals called neurotrophins, which support the survival and growth of brain cells. Additionally, exercise has been shown to reduce inflammation and oxidative stress, both of which can negatively impact cognitive function.

Enhancing Mental Clarity, Focus, and Creativity through Exercise

Exercise not only improves physical health but also enhances mental clarity, focus, and creativity. When you engage in physical activity, your brain releases endorphins, neurotransmitters that promote a positive mood and reduce stress and anxiety. This boost in mood can enhance mental clarity and focus, making it easier to concentrate on tasks and make sound decisions. Moreover, exercise has been shown to increase the production of brain-derived neurotrophic factor (BDNF), a protein that supports the growth of new neurons and improves cognitive function. By incorporating regular exercise into your routine, you can experience heightened mental acuity and unleash your creativity.

Strategies for Incorporating Mindfulness and Stress Management into Your Fitness Routine

In addition to physical exercise, incorporating mindfulness and stress management techniques into your fitness routine can further enhance your mental performance. Mindfulness involves being fully present in the moment and non-judgmentally aware of your thoughts, feelings, and sensations. Practicing mindfulness during exercise can help you focus on the task at hand, increase self-awareness, and reduce stress. Consider incorporating activities such as yoga, tai chi, or mindful walking into your fitness routine to cultivate a sense of calm and mental clarity.

Stress management is also crucial for optimizing mental performance. Exercise itself is a powerful stress reliever, as it reduces levels of stress hormones and promotes the release of endorphins. However, incorporating additional stress management techniques can further enhance the benefits. Consider integrating practices such as meditation, deep breathing exercises, or journaling into your fitness routine to effectively manage stress and promote mental well-being.

Creating a Balanced Fitness and Mental Performance Routine

To create a balanced fitness and mental performance routine, it's important to prioritize both physical exercise and mental well-being. Aim for a combination of cardiovascular exercises, strength training, and flexibility exercises to improve physical fitness. Dedicate regular time to engage in activities that promote mindfulness and stress management, such as yoga or meditation. Consider setting aside specific periods for mental performance activities, such as problem-solving exercises or creative pursuits, to enhance cognitive function.

Remember to listen to your body and make adjustments as needed. Rest and recovery are essential for both physical and mental well-being, so incorporate rest days into your routine to prevent burnout and optimize performance.

Conclusion

Physical fitness and mental performance are deeply interconnected. By understanding the correlation between physical exercise and cognitive function, you can leverage the power of fitness to enhance your mental clarity, focus, and creativity. Incorporating mindfulness and stress management techniques into your fitness routine further promotes mental well-being. By creating a balanced fitness and mental performance routine, you can optimize your overall well-being as an entrepreneur and achieve peak performance in both your personal and professional life. Embrace the synergy between fitness and mental performance and unlock your full potential.

6

Nutrition for Optimal Performance

In this chapter, we will explore the vital role of nutrition in supporting both physical and mental well-being. As an entrepreneur, it is crucial to fuel your body and mind with the right nutrients to maximize your performance and achieve success. We will delve into the significance of nutrition, discuss how to tailor your diet to support entrepreneurial endeavors and provide practical tips for meal planning, hydration, and supplementation for busy individuals. By prioritizing your nutrition, you can optimize your energy levels, enhance cognitive function, and promote overall health and vitality.

Understanding the Role of Nutrition in Supporting Physical and Mental Well-Being

Nutrition plays a fundamental role in supporting physical and mental well-being. It provides the necessary nutrients to fuel bodily functions, repair tissues, and promote optimal health. Adequate nutrition is crucial for maintaining energy levels, enhancing cognitive function, managing stress, and supporting immune function. By adopting a balanced and nutrient-dense diet, you can lay the foundation for optimal physical and mental performance.

Tailoring Your Diet to Fuel Entrepreneurial Success

As an entrepreneur, your dietary choices should align with your goals and lifestyle. Consider the following principles to tailor your diet for optimal performance:

1. Balanced Macro nutrients: Include a balance of carbohydrates, proteins, and healthy fats in your meals to provide sustained energy and support various bodily functions.
2. Nutrient-Dense Foods: Prioritize whole, unprocessed foods that are rich in vitamins, minerals, and antioxidants. Include plenty of fruits, vegetables, lean proteins, whole grains, and healthy fats in your diet.
3. Mindful Eating: Practice mindful eating by paying attention to your hunger and fullness cues, and savoring your meals. Avoid mindless snacking or eating while distracted.
4. Hydration: Stay adequately hydrated by drinking water throughout the day. Proper hydration supports cognitive function, digestion, and overall health.

Meal Planning, Hydration, and Supplementation Tips for Busy Individuals

For busy entrepreneurs, effective meal planning, hydration, and supplementation can make a significant difference in maintaining optimal nutrition. Consider the following tips:

1. Meal Planning: Plan your meals in advance to ensure you have nutritious options readily available. Prepare and pack meals and snacks to avoid relying on unhealthy fast food or processed options.
2. Batch Cooking: Save time by preparing larger quantities of meals and storing them for future consumption. This approach allows you to have nutritious meals ready to eat even during busy days.

3. Smart Snacking: Keep a stash of healthy snacks, such as nuts, seeds, fruits, or protein bars, to fuel you throughout the day and prevent energy crashes.

4. Hydration Strategies: Set reminders to drink water regularly and keep a water bottle with you at all times. Infuse water with fruits or herbs for added flavor and encourage hydration.

5. Nutritional Supplementation: Consider incorporating supplements, such as a multivitamin, omega-3 fatty acids, or probiotics, into your routine to fill potential nutrient gaps. Consult with a healthcare professional to determine your specific needs.

6. Mindful Eating Breaks: Take regular breaks during work to have focused, mindful meals. Step away from your desk, savor your food, and give your body and mind a chance to recharge.

7. Seek Professional Guidance: If you have specific dietary needs or goals, consult a registered dietitian or nutritionist who can provide personalized recommendations and guidance.

Conclusion

Nutrition is a cornerstone of optimal physical and mental performance for entrepreneurs. By understanding the importance of nutrition, tailoring your diet to support your goals, and implementing effective strategies like meal planning, hydration, and supplementation, you can fuel your body and mind for entrepreneurial success. Prioritize nutrient-dense foods, practice mindful eating, and seek professional guidance when necessary. Remember that your nutrition is a key component of your overall well-being and can significantly impact your productivity, focus, and overall health as you navigate the entrepreneurial journey.

7

Overcoming Fitness Plateaus and Challenges

In this chapter, we will explore the common obstacles that individuals face in maintaining a consistent fitness routine and achieving their fitness goals. We will discuss strategies for overcoming fitness plateaus, avoiding burnout, and embracing a sustainable, long-term approach to fitness. By understanding and addressing these challenges, you can maintain your motivation, break through plateaus, and achieve lasting success in your fitness journey.

Identifying Common Obstacles in Maintaining a Consistent Fitness Routine

Maintaining a consistent fitness routine can be challenging due to various obstacles. Some common hurdles include:

1. Lack of Time: Busy schedules and competing priorities can make it difficult to find time for exercise.
2. Lack of Motivation: It's natural to experience periods of low motivation, especially when faced with setbacks or plateaus.
3. Physical Fatigue: Overtraining, inadequate recovery, or physical fatigue can hinder progress and increase the risk of injury.

23

4. Monotony and Boredom: Doing the same exercises or routines repetitively can lead to boredom and a lack of enjoyment.

Strategies for Breaking Through Plateaus and Avoiding Burnout

To overcome plateaus and avoid burnout, consider implementing the following strategies:

1. Set New Goals: Set specific, measurable, achievable, relevant, and time-bound (SMART) goals to provide direction and motivation.
2. Vary Your Routine: Incorporate variety into your workouts by trying new exercises, training methods, or fitness classes. This can help prevent boredom and challenge your body in different ways.
3. Cross-Train: Engage in different types of exercise, such as strength training, cardiovascular activities, and flexibility exercises, to work for different muscle groups and prevent overuse injuries.
4. Track Your Progress: Keep a record of your workouts, including sets, reps, and weights used. Tracking your progress can help you identify areas of improvement and provide a sense of accomplishment.
5. Seek Support and Accountability: Enlist the support of a workout buddy, join fitness communities, or hire a personal trainer to provide accountability, motivation, and guidance.
6. Rest and Recovery: Prioritize rest and recovery days to allow your body to repair and recharge. Adequate sleep, proper nutrition, and active recovery techniques can help prevent burnout and optimize performance.

Embracing a Sustainable, Long-Term Approach to Fitness

To maintain a sustainable, long-term approach to fitness, consider the following:

1. Consistency over Intensity: Focus on consistency in your workouts rather than constantly pushing for maximum intensity. Consistent effort over time yields better results and reduces the risk of burnout or injury.

2. Prioritize Self-Care: Take care of your overall well-being by incorporating stress management techniques, adequate sleep, and healthy eating habits into your lifestyle.

3. Listen to Your Body: Pay attention to your body's signals and adjust your training accordingly. Allow for recovery when needed and modify your workouts to accommodate any limitations or injuries.

4. Celebrate Small Wins: Acknowledge and celebrate your progress, no matter how small. Recognizing your achievements along the way can boost motivation and keep you on track.

5. Enjoy the Process: Find enjoyment and fulfillment in the journey itself rather than solely focusing on the end result. Embrace the positive physical and mental changes that exercise brings to your life.

Conclusion

Overcoming fitness plateaus and challenges is an integral part of maintaining a consistent and successful fitness routine. By identifying common obstacles, implementing strategies to break through plateaus and avoid burnout, and embracing a sustainable, long-term approach to fitness, you can overcome hurdles and achieve lasting results. Remember that fitness is a lifelong journey, and by staying adaptable, motivated, and committed, you can navigate any challenges that come your way.

9 798395 827838